SOLUTION TO PRESSURE ULCER

EVERYTHING YOU NEED TO KNOW ABOUT PRESSURE ULCERS: A STEP-BY-STEP GUIDE

DR. PETER .DYLAN

Table of Contents

- CHAPTER ONE 2
- INTRODUCTION TO PRESSURE ULCER 2
  - DEFINITION OF PRESSURE ULCERS 7
  - SIGNIFICANCE OF DISCUSSING PRESSURE ULCERS 10
- CHAPTER TWO 17
  - CAUSES OF PRESSURE ULCERS 17
  - RISK ELEMENTS FOR DEVELOPING PRESSURE ULCERS 22
- CHAPTER THREE 30
  - SIGNS AND SYMPTOMS OF PRESSURE ULCERS 30
  - DESCRIPTION OF THE SORTS OF PRESSURE ULCERS 37
  - PREVENTION OF PRESSURE ULCERS 42
- CHAPTER FOUR 47
  - STRATEGIES FOR PREVENTING PRESSURE ULCERS 47
  - EXPLANATION OF THE EXCLUSIVE REMEDY ALTERNATIVES FOR PRESSURE ULCERS 52
- CHAPTER FIVE 60
  - COMPLICATIONS OF PRESSURE ULCERS 60
  - CONCLUSION OF PRESSURE ULCERS 71
- THE END 77

CHAPTER ONE

INTRODUCTION TO PRESSURE ULCER

Pressure ulcers are a common healthcare problem that affects humans of every age, from toddlers to older people. Those wounds can be painful, brutal, leading to extreme complications if left untreated. If you or a loved one has ever suffered from a pressure ulcer, you know how hard it could be to manage these wounds. We will discuss strain ulcers, their causes, signs and symptoms, and remedy alternatives. Whether you are a healthcare professional or a person who the aid of strain ulcers has personally impacted, this will provide useful statistics on this essential subject matter. So, let's dive into the sector of pressure ulcers and learn more about this commonplace healthcare difficulty.

Stress ulcers, also known as bedsores, are an unusual but regularly misunderstood scientific circumstance that can have an effect on anyone with limited mobility. Whether you or a loved one has lately been recognized with a strain ulcer or needs to analyze more about this condition we can explore strain ulcers and their reasons, symptoms, and remedy options. You will better understand what stress ulcers are and how to prevent them from taking place in the first place. So, without further ado, let's dive right in!

Pressure ulcers are a commonplace and sometimes serious scientific situation that affects people of every age. These painful sores can broaden while someone remains in one position for too long, damaging the pores and skin. If left untreated, pressure ulcers can result in infection, tissue damage, or even the loss of life. But, with the right care and prevention techniques, pressure ulcers can be avoided. we can explore the causes, signs, and remedies of strain ulcers to help you better recognize this situation and find a way to prevent it. Pressure ulcers are a commonplace hassle that affects many people, especially those who are bedridden or wheelchair-bound. Those wounds may be painful, debilitating, and, in severe cases, life-threatening. Despite their prevalence, pressure ulcers are frequently misunderstood and neglected. We will explore the topic of strain ulcers, delving into their reasons, signs and symptoms, prevention, and treatment alternatives. Whether you have experienced a pressure ulcer or are interested in learning more about this situation, we intend to offer complete statistics that allow you to better understand and control strain ulcers.

Stress ulcers, also known as bedsores, are common among folks who are bedridden or wheelchair-bound for prolonged periods. Those painful and regularly debilitating wounds can be frustrating to address, but with the proper care and treatment, they can be averted and treated correctly. we will explore the subject of pressure ulcers in detail, discussing their reasons, signs and symptoms, and remedy options. Whether or not you or a loved one are at risk for stress ulcers or want to research more about this not-unusual clinical situation, this publication will provide valuable insights and statistics.

DEFINITION OF PRESSURE ULCERS

Pressure ulcers, also called bedsores or strain sores, are a commonplace and doubtlessly serious health hassle affecting many patients, particularly those who spend lengthy time on a mattress or in a wheelchair. In reality, pressure ulcers are anticipated to affect up to 3 million people in the United States every 12 months. Pressure ulcers result from prolonged pressure on the skin and underlying tissues that can cause harm, irritation, and tissue demise. This pressure can result from various factors, including immobility, terrible vitamins, friction, and moisture. The most common areas where strain ulcers develop are over bony prominences of the hips, ankles, heels, and tailbone.

The development of pressure ulcers can be prevented with the right care and interest. Normal turning and repositioning of patients, along with cautious skin care and management of moisture, can help reduce the hazard of strain ulcers. Further, the right nutrients and hydration are critical to maintaining wholesome pores and skin and stopping stress ulcers.

The symptoms of pressure ulcers can vary depending on the severity of the damage. Early symptoms can also include redness or discoloration of the skin, swelling, and tenderness. Because the harm progresses, the pores and skin may also smash down and shape an open sore that may emerge as infected and cause more severe headaches.

The treatment of stress ulcers depends on the severity of the injury. Moderate cases may be handled with wound care and infection control, while more severe cases may require surgical intervention or specialized wound care products. In all instances, early detection and treatment are vital to preventing similar injuries and complications.

pressure ulcers are an extreme and commonplace fitness hassle that can have widespread consequences for patients and caregivers. By taking steps to prevent strain ulcers and identifying and treating them early, we will help ensure first-class viable results for patients and minimize the effect of this circumstance on our healthcare gadget. If you or a loved one is at risk for pressure ulcers, speak to your healthcare company about prevention and treatment options.

SIGNIFICANCE OF DISCUSSING PRESSURE ULCERS

Pressure ulcers, also known as bedsores, are a common situation affecting thousands and thousands of humans worldwide. These ulcers may be sufferers' main source of discomfort and pain and may cause severe headaches if left untreated. While stress ulcers are often related to elderly sufferers or people with mobility troubles, they can occur in anyone immobile or bedridden for a prolonged period. we will discuss the importance of discussing stress ulcers and why it's important for sufferers and caregivers alike to be aware of this condition. Stress ulcers are caused by prolonged pressure at the pores, skin, and underlying tissues, which could occur while someone is immobile or bedridden for prolonged periods. This pressure can cause damage to the pores, skin, and tissues, leading to the improvement of ulcers. Further to immobility, different factors that could contribute to improving stress ulcers consist of poor nutrition, incontinence, and positive clinical situations, including diabetes.

While pressure ulcers may appear minor, they could have severe consequences if left untreated. In excessive instances, stress ulcers can result in infections, sepsis, and other lifestyle-threatening complications. Moreover, pressure ulcers can be extraordinarily painful and drastically lessen a patient's quality of life.

Fortuitously, some steps may be taken to save you and treat strain ulcers. Patients at risk for developing strain ulcers must be repositioned often and provided with stress-relieving devices, including cushions or mattresses. The right nutrients and hydration are also vital for stopping strain ulcers, preserving proper hygiene and keeping the pores and skin smooth and dry.

If a pressure ulcer expands, seeking treatment as quickly as possible is crucial. The remedy can also involve cleaning the wound and applying dressings or topical medicinal drugs to promote restoration. In more severe cases, a surgical procedure may be necessary to do away with broken tissue and facilitate recovery.

Notwithstanding the critical outcomes that can result from pressure ulcers, many patients and caregivers are unaware of this condition or do not take it seriously enough. By discussing stress ulcers and raising awareness of this circumstance, we can assist in preventing the improvement of strain ulcers and ensure that sufferers get the care and treatment they want.

Pressure ulcers are a critical situation that may have large effects if left untreated. By discussing pressure ulcers and taking steps to prevent and treat them, we can help sufferers acquire the care they want and may keep their great lives. If you or someone you know is at risk for growing strain ulcers, speak to a healthcare provider about how to save you and treat this condition.

Pressure ulcers, called bedsores, are a common and preventable circumstance impacting millions of humans worldwide. These sores arise while the pores, skin, and underlying tissue are damaged because of extended stress and the absence of blood flow to the region. Strain ulcers may be a massive trouble for sufferers who're bedridden, wheelchair-certain, or have restricted mobility and might cause severe headaches such as infections, sepsis, and even death. Discussing stress ulcers with your loved ones and healthcare providers is vital because prevention is fundamental. The first step in preventing strain ulcers is to become aware of those at risk. Older patients, have restrained mobility, or are bedridden have a higher chance of developing strain ulcers. As soon as the problem is recognized, preventative measures can be taken, including repositioning every few hours, using specialized cushions and mattresses to distribute stress, and keeping the pores and skin clean and dry.

Early detection and remedy are also critical in preventing pressure ulcers from worsening. Signs of pressure ulcers include redness, swelling, and skin that feel warmer or cooler to touch than surrounding areas. If you are aware of any of those signs and symptoms, searching for clinical interest at once is critical.

By discussing pressure ulcers with your family and healthcare vendors, you can work together to develop an effective prevention and remedy plan. This can encompass precise care instructions, consisting of how regularly to reposition and turn the affected person and using a specialized device. Schooling on the right vitamins and hydration is essential for the most effective pores and skin health.

Further to preventing and treating pressure ulcers, discussing this situation can also help raise awareness and decrease stigma. Patients may feel ashamed or embarrassed to have stress ulcers. Still, it is important to consider that that is a common circumstance that could appear to everybody with restricted mobility. By openly discussing strain ulcers, we can reduce the stigma related to this situation and promote a compassionate and understanding approach to healthcare. Discussing stress ulcers is important for patients, caregivers, and healthcare providers. We can reduce the occurrence and severity of strain ulcers by figuring out the ones at risk, taking preventative measures, and looking for early remedies

CHAPTER TWO

CAUSES OF PRESSURE ULCERS

Pressure ulcers, referred to as bedsores or pressure sores, are a common situation affecting millions worldwide Extended strain, friction, and shear forces causes stress ulcers. Those forces can cause damage to the pores, skin, and underlying tissues, leading to the formation of an ulcer. Stress ulcers can occur in all and sundry, but they are more common in immobile or with a medical condition that impacts mobility. we will discuss the reasons for stress ulcers and how to prevent them.

Prolonged strain

Extended pressure is the most common reason for strain ulcers. When someone is immobile for a prolonged period, the weight of their body places pressure on positive areas of the frame, consisting of the hips, heels, and tailbone This stress can cause the pores, skin, and underlying tissues to end up compressed, leading to a loss of blood flow and oxygen to the region.

Without the right blood flow and oxygen, the pores, skin, and tissues can start to break down, forming an ulcer. Folks who are bedridden or restricted to a wheelchair are at the very best risk for growing pressure ulcers because of extended strain.

Friction

Friction is the other purpose of stress ulcers. Friction occurs while the pores and skin rub against a floor, causing small tears and harm to the skin. When combined with extended stress, friction can cause pressure ulcers.

Friction may be caused by a diffusion of factors, including difficult mattress sheets, poorly equipped clothing, or sliding down in a chair or wheelchair.

Shear Forces

Shear forces occur while the pores and skin move in a single direction simultaneously as the underlying tissues flow in some other direction. This can cause damage to the skin and underlying tissues, leading to the formation of an ulcer Shear forces are frequently visible in those who are bedridden or restricted to a wheelchair. When someone is repositioned on a mattress or transferred from a wheelchair to a mattress, the skin and tissues may be pulled in specific directions, causing shear forces.

Prevention

Stopping strain ulcers is crucial to preserving the fitness and well-being of those who are bedridden or have confined mobility. Here are some tips for preventing pressure ulcers:

- Repositioning: frequent repositioning is important for stopping strain ulcers. This may be accomplished by changing positions each hour or using a stress-relieving mattress or cushion.
- Pores and skin care: preserving and keeping the skin moisturized is crucial to preventing stress ulcers. Avoid using hot water and harsh soaps; use moderate cleaning soap and warm water.
- Nutrition: A well-balanced food regimen is crucial to retaining healthy skin and stopping strain ulcers. Ensure that people at risk for pressure ulcers have a weight-

reduction plan rich in protein, nutrients, and minerals.

- exercising is critical to maintaining healthy skin and stopping stress ulcers. Even simple exercises, stretching, and range of motion physical games can help save you from stress ulcers.

Strain ulcers are a common circumstance that can cause huge pain and soreness for people who are bedridden or have constrained mobility. Expertise in the causes of stress ulcers and taking preventative measures is vital to maintaining the fitness and well-being of people at risk. With the pointers mentioned, you can help prevent the formation of stress ulcers and ensure that people with restricted mobility have healthy skin.

RISK ELEMENTS FOR DEVELOPING PRESSURE ULCERS

Pressure ulcers, additionally called bedsores, are a commonplace hassle for those limited to a mattress or a wheelchair for extended periods. Those painful and potentially dangerous sores are caused by extended stress on the pores, skin, and underlying tissue, which could damage blood vessels and nerves. Even though everyone can develop pressure ulcers, positive danger elements increase the chance of their development. Age is certainly one of the most important risk factors for strain ulcers. As we age, our skin will become thinner and much less elastic, putting it at greater risk of harm. Older adults also have a higher chance of clinical situations that can contribute to improving stress ulcers, along with diabetes and stream problems.

Folks with motionless or constrained mobility are also at elevated risk for pressure ulcers. This consists of those who are bedridden or confined to a wheelchair and those who've suffered a spinal cord injury or have a neuromuscular disorder. While the body performs a single function for a prolonged time frame, strain is placed on certain regions of the skin, which may cause the improvement of pressure ulcers.

Bad nutrition can also increase the risk of strain ulcers. A diet lacking in protein, vitamin C, and other vital nutrients can cause the skin to emerge as weak and more prone to harm. Dehydration can increase the danger of stress ulcers, as it may cause the skin to emerge as dry and extra at risk of harm.

Different elements that can contribute to the development of stress ulcers encompass obesity, smoking, and positive clinical conditions, which include peripheral vascular sickness or congestive coronary heart failure. Similarly, individuals with a history of pressure ulcers are in increased danger of developing or developing them once more.

Preventing strain ulcers is key to ward off the aches, pains, pains, and potential health headaches that could arise from their development. This consists of preserving accurate skin hygiene, keeping skin dry and clean, and changing positions often to reduce strain on any frame location. Proper nutrition and hydration are also vital for preserving healthy pores and skin.

If you or a loved one is in danger of developing strain ulcers, it's critical to take steps to save them. By learning about the chance elements and taking appropriate measures to reduce them, you may help help protect your pores and skin and avoid the aches and headaches of stress ulcers.

Strain ulcers, referred to as bedsores or pressure sores, are a common trouble for folks who are bedridden or spend long time in a wheelchair. They arise when strain is applied to the pores, skin, and gentle tissue over bony regions of the body, inflicting damage to the underlying tissue. we can discuss the hazard factors for growing stress ulcers.

1. Immobility: one of the number one threat factors for growing stress ulcers is

immobility. While someone is bedridden or confined to a wheelchair, they may be much more likely to develop pressure ulcers because they're unable to change positions often enough to alleviate stress on certain regions of the body. This loss of mobility can cause extended strain on the pores, skin, and soft tissue, which can cause damage over the years.

2. Age: As we age, our pores and skin become thinner and much less elastic, making us more susceptible to pressure ulcers. Moreover, older adults may additionally have medical situations that restrict their mobility or motivate them to spend more time in bed or in a wheelchair, further increasing their chance of developing strain ulcers.

3. Negative nutrients: A healthy weight-reduction plan is important for retaining

wholesome pores and skin. When someone's food regimen is lacking in vital vitamins and nutrients, their pores and skin may additionally end up more susceptible to damage, including strain ulcers. Additionally, people who are malnourished may also have weakened immune systems, making it harder for their bodies to fight off infections that may expand into pressure ulcers.

4. Incontinence: incontinent individuals, meaning they're unable to govern their bladder or bowels, are at an elevated risk of developing pressure ulcers. That is because the skin inside the location across the genitals and buttocks can emerge irritated and broken from prolonged exposure to urine or feces.

5. Continual scientific conditions: people with continual scientific situations,

including diabetes or vascular sickness, may be at a higher risk of developing pressure ulcers. Those situations can affect blood and oxygen flow to the skin and smooth tissue, making it more difficult for the frame to heal and increasing the threat of growing pressure ulcers.

6. Smoking: Smoking can affect the pores and skin in some ways, including decreasing blood waft to the pores and skin and making it more vulnerable to harm. Smoke individuals may be at increased risk of developing pressure ulcers and other skin conditions.

Stress ulcers are not uncommon trouble for folks who are bedridden or spend lengthy intervals of time in a wheelchair. Several factors can increase a person's chance of developing strain ulcers, including immobility, age, negative nutrition, incontinence, persistent scientific conditions, and smoking. With expertise in these hazard factors, humans can take steps to prevent pressure ulcers from growing and defend their pores, skin, and usual fitness.

CHAPTER THREE

SIGNS AND SYMPTOMS OF PRESSURE ULCERS

Pressure ulcers, also called bedsores or strain sores, are accidents that occur at the pores, skin, and underlying tissues due to extended pressure on a selected body place. They typically broaden to include those bedridden or motionless for prolonged durations, including those in nursing homes or hospitals. Stress ulcers may be painful and tough to manage, and if left untreated, they can result in critical headaches. we will discuss the signs of strain ulcers and what to do if you suspect you or a loved one has an advanced one. The primary symptom of a strain ulcer is typically redness or discoloration of the skin. The affected area may be warm to the touch and feel tender or itchy. This is typically the first sign that a strain ulcer is developing, and it's critical to do so at this stage to prevent the ulcer from worsening. The skin may become blistered or open as the pressure ulcer progresses, exposing underlying tissues. The wound may appear as a shallow crater or a deep, open sore. The pores and skin across the ulcer may be discolored or have a different texture than the encircling skin. The affected location can also have a nasty smell or discharge.

In severe instances, stress ulcers can extend deep into the underlying tissues, affecting muscles, bones, and joints. This may bring about considerable pain and a lack of features. Insufficient strain ulcers can cause serious headaches, infections, and sepsis.

If you suspect that you or a cherished one has developed a stress ulcer, it's essential to seek medical attention immediately. Your healthcare provider can verify the severity of the ulcer and suggest a precise treatment. The remedy may include wound care, antibiotics to prevent or deal with infections, and pain control.

Preventing pressure ulcers is important, especially for bedridden or motionless patients. It's far more critical to trade roles regularly and use specialized cushions or pads to reduce strain on bony regions. Precise skin care and the right cleaning and moisturizing can also improve strain ulcers.

Pressure ulcers are a serious and sometimes painful circumstance that may develop in people who are bedridden or immobile for prolonged intervals. The symptoms of strain ulcers include redness, discoloration, blisters, open sores, and foul odors or discharge. If you suspect that you or a loved one has developed a strain ulcer, seek medical attention immediately. Prevention is prime, and taking steps to reduce strain on bony regions and maintain proper skin care can help prevent pressure ulcers.

Pressure ulcers, also called bedsores or pressure sores, are a commonplace hassle for people limited to a mattress or wheelchair for prolonged periods. They're due to extended stress on the skin and underlying tissue, harming the pores, skin, and underlying tissue. Strain ulcers may be painful and hard to deal with, and they can even lead to critical infections if left untreated. We'll talk about the signs and symptoms of stress ulcers so you can become aware of them early and search for a remedy.

1. Redness or discoloration

The first sign of a pressure ulcer is usually redness or discoloration of the skin. This discoloration can be red, pink, or blue and may feel warm. The skin may also feel soft or painful and may be itchy. Talk to your healthcare company if you observe any redness or discoloration of your pores and skin, particularly if it doesn't go away after changing positions.

2. Swelling

As pressure ulcers develop, they can cause swelling inside the affected region. This swelling may be mild or excessive, making it hard to transport or use the affected limb. If you notice swelling in a place and are experiencing redness or discoloration, or if you are experiencing pain or soreness, look for clinical interest right away.

3. Open sores

As strain ulcers develop, they could cause open sores or wounds. These sores can be shallow or deep and may be observed via drainage or fluid buildup. If you observe any open sores, particularly those that aren't healing or are followed by different signs, seek medical attention immediately.

4. Numbness or tingling

As pressure ulcers progress, they can cause numbness or tingling in the affected region. This may be observed through a loss of sensation or a feeling of pins and needles. If you observe any numbness or tingling on your skin, particularly inside the areas where you're experiencing redness or discoloration, seek clinical attention immediately.

5. Foul scent

As strain ulcers progress, they can become infected and emit a foul odor. This odor may be great even before you notice any other signs. If you notice any unusual odors, specifically those coming from an area experiencing redness or discoloration, search for medical information immediately.

Strain ulcers are a severe issue that can cause pain, ache, and even severe infections if left untreated. If you notice any of the signs referred to above, ensure you are trying to find scientific attention immediately. Early treatment can help prevent headaches and enhance your general health and well-being.

DESCRIPTION OF THE SORTS OF PRESSURE ULCERS

Pressure ulcers, also called bed sores or strain sores, are a common fitness hassle that impacts people restricted to a mattress or a wheelchair for a prolonged period. Those ulcers result from extended stress on a selected part of the frame, which may result in the breakdown of skin and underlying tissues. Pressure ulcers are categorized into one-of-a-kind ranges primarily based on their severity, and information about those stages can assist individuals and healthcare specialists in preventing and treating these painful wounds. Degree 1 stress ulcers:

Stage 1 pressure ulcers are the mildest form of strain ulcers. They may be characterized by a reddened area on the skin that does not blanch when pressed. This level indicates harm to the skin and underlying tissues, but the harm has no longer broken the pores and skin. Level 1 strain ulcers are usually handled by removing the strain and keeping the region clean and dry.

Degree 2 stresses ulcers:

Degree 2 strain ulcers are characterized by a shallow open wound that resembles a blister or a shallow crater. The wound may be purple or crimson and can have a few fluid drainages. The skin and underlying tissues are broken at this level, and the wound can be painful. The remedy for degree 2 strain ulcers includes:

- Removing pressure from the vicinity.
- Keeping the place clean and dry.

- Using dressings to protect the wound.

Degree 3 pressure ulcers:

Stage three stress ulcers are characterized by a deep wound that extends through the skin and into the underlying tissues. The wound may also seem like a crater and may have some yellow or useless tissue. At this level, the wound is painful and can be inflamed.

The remedy for level 3 pressure ulcers includes:

- Removing strain from the vicinity.
- Cleansing the wound.
- Removing useless tissue.
- Applying dressings to shield the wound.

Level 4 pressure ulcers:

Level 4 stress ulcers are the most extreme form of stress ulcer. In this stage, the wound extends through the pores and skin into the underlying tissues, muscle mass, and bones. The wound may also appear like a deep crater with a few useless tissues. To this degree, the wound could be very painful and have an excessive chance of contamination. The remedy for level four pressure ulcers consists of removing strain from the place, cleaning the wound, removing dead tissue, and applying dressings to guard the wound. Surgery may be required in extreme instances to remove the damaged tissue and promote healing.

Prevention is key to fending off strain ulcers. Ensure that individuals restrained to a bed or wheelchair is repositioned regularly and that their skin is kept clean and dry. Also, ensure they consume a wholesome weight-reduction plan and get enough fluids to keep their pores and skin healthy.

Pressure ulcers are a commonplace health hassle that can be avoided and treated properly. Expertise in the specific stages of stress ulcers can help individuals and healthcare experts prevent and treat those painful wounds. Prevention is key to preventing strain ulcers, and taking vital steps can ensure that individuals restrained to a bed or wheelchair is secure and healthy.

PREVENTION OF PRESSURE ULCERS

Pressure ulcers, additionally known as bedsores or stress sores, are a commonplace problem in individuals who are bedridden or have restricted mobility. Those sores arise from extended strain on the pores and skin and may be extraordinarily painful and debilitating. Strain ulcers can also cause serious infections and might even be life-threatening in intense cases. But the appropriate information is that stress ulcers may be avoided with proper care and interest. We can discuss the prevention of strain ulcers and the steps you could take to keep yourself or your family secure from this painful circumstance.

1. Flow often.

Moving regularly is one of the most important steps in stopping stress ulcers. If you or your loved one is bedridden, change positions every two hours to alleviate pressure on certain regions of the frame. If you are in a wheelchair, shift your weight every 15 minutes. This will help promote blood flow and prevent the formation of pressure ulcers.

2. Maintain smooth and dry skin.

Keeping the skin clean and dry is also important for stopping stress ulcers. Moisture can increase the risk of pores and skin breakdown, so it's vital to dry the pores and skin very well after bathing or using the toilet. Make certain to use mild soaps and avoid scrubbing the skin too hard, which can cause irritation and damage.

3. Use assistive surfaces

Using assistive surfaces, which include special cushions or mattresses, can also help prevent stress ulcers. These surfaces help distribute strain evenly and decrease the hazard of pores and skin breakdown. Communicate to your healthcare provider what form of support surface is probably first-class for you or the one you love.

4. Maintain a wholesome food plan.

A healthy weight loss plan rich in protein and nutrients can also help prevent pressure ulcers. Protein is important for tissue repair and regeneration, so lean meats, fish, eggs, and dairy products should be included in your weight loss plan. Fruits and veggies are also crucial for basic fitness and can provide essential vitamins and minerals, which are crucial for pores and skin fitness.

5. Stay hydrated.

Staying hydrated is also crucial to stopping stress ulcers. Dehydration can cause dry, cracked pores and skin that is more susceptible to pores and skin breakdown. Ensure you drink fluids for the day, preferably water, to keep your pores and skin wholesome and hydrated.

6. Get ordinary check-ups

Normal tests in the United States of America with your healthcare issuer are also essential in stopping pressure ulcers. Your healthcare provider can display your pores and skin health and recommend stopping stress ulcers. They can also offer treatment if a strain ulcer does increase.

Pressure ulcers are a critical problem for people with restricted mobility, but they may be averted with the right care and attention. By following those simple steps, you can help keep yourself or your family secure from the pain and discomfort of pressure ulcers. Consider moving frequently, keeping skin clean and dry, using support surfaces, maintaining a wholesome diet, staying hydrated, and getting ordinary checkups. Live wholesomely and happily!

CHAPTER FOUR

STRATEGIES FOR PREVENTING PRESSURE ULCERS

Pressure ulcers, also known as bedsores or pressure sores, are a common problem for folks who are limited to a bed or a wheelchair for prolonged intervals of time. These sores may be painful, slow to heal, and even result in extreme infections. However, some techniques may be employed to prevent the development of stress ulcers in the first place. we can discover some of these strategies that can help can help you or a loved one avoid strain ulcers.

1. Change positions regularly.

One of the most critical techniques for stopping pressure ulcers is regularly changing roles. This indicates shifting your weight every couple of hours if you are in a bed or repositioning yourself every 15 minutes if you are in a wheelchair. The aim is to alleviate stress in certain areas of the body, including the hips, buttocks, and heels, the most common locations for pressure ulcers.

2. Use specialized cushions and mattresses.

effective way to prevent pressure ulcers is to use specialized cushions and mattresses that might be designed to distribute stress evenly throughout the frame. Those items can be purchased online or via medical supply stores and can be utilized in beds, wheelchairs, and different seating arrangements.

3. Maintain skin easy and dry.dry.

Keeping the skin smooth and dry is likewise essential for preventing pressure ulcers. This indicates taking ordinary baths or showers, using mild cleaning soap, and patting the pores and skin dry with a gentle towel. Using moisturizer can also help preserve the skin's suppleness and prevent it from becoming dry and cracked.

4. Devour a balanced eating regimen.

A balanced eating regimen rich in protein, nutrients, and minerals is important for preserving healthy pores and skin. The pores and skin need these vitamins to repair themselves and withstand contamination. If you or a loved one has problems consuming, speak to a medical doctor or dietician about ensuring you get the necessary vitamins.

5. Exercise often.

Everyday exercise is vital for preserving a healthy body and preventing stress ulcers. This may encompass easy sports such as stretching, variety-of-movement physical activities, and wheelchair physical activities. Speak to a physical therapist or physician about high-quality exercises for you or a loved one.

6. Keep away from friction and shear.

Friction and shear can cause stress ulcers to increase quickly. Friction happens while the skin rubs against clothing or bedding, while shear occurs when the skin is pulled in unique directions or when someone slides down in a bed. To prevent friction and shear, use a boost sheet while transferring a person from a bed to a wheelchair and avoid dragging or pulling the individual across surfaces.

7. Monitor pores and skin conditions.

Eventually, it's critical to monitor the pores and skin for any signs and symptoms of pressure ulcers. This consists of redness, swelling, and tenderness, which are the primary symptoms of a stress ulcer. If you know of any of these signs, communicate with a physician or nurse immediately.

Pressure ulcers may be an extreme problem for people confined to a mattress or a wheelchair. But, by employing those strategies, you or a loved one can lessen the threat of growing stress ulcers and keep wholesome pores and skin. Remember to exchange roles frequently, use specialized cushions and mattresses, preserve skin clean and dry, eat a balanced food plan, exercise frequently, keep away from friction and shear, and monitor skin conditions. Following these tips can prevent pressure ulcers and enjoy better fitness and well-being.

EXPLANATION OF THE EXCLUSIVE REMEDY ALTERNATIVES FOR PRESSURE ULCERS

Pressure ulcers, referred to as bedsores, are a form of harm that happens when the skin and underlying tissue are compressed over a protracted period. Those injuries are most commonly visible in those restrained to a bed or wheelchair for an extended period, and they could cause critical health headaches if left untreated. Happily, there are several special remedy alternatives to be had for individuals who are suffering from strain ulcers. One of the most common remedies for stress ulcers is using dressings. Dressings are applied to the wound to help keep it smooth and prevent further harm to the skin and underlying tissue. Several extraordinary forms of dressings can be used for strain ulcers, along with hydrocolloid dressings, foam dressings, and alginate dressings. Each dressing has its blessings and disadvantages, so it's far more important to work with a healthcare issuer to decide which dressing is right for your situation.

Another common alternative remedy for pressure ulcers is the use of topical drugs. Topical retailers are creams, ointments, or gels that might be applied immediately to the wound. Those agents can help to lessen pain, inflammation, and infection, and they can also promote recovery. Some of the most commonly used topical marketers for pressure ulcers include antimicrobial retailers, such as silver sulfadiazine, and boom factors, including recombinant human epidermal increase factor.

A surgical operation may be vital for more severe instances of strain ulcers. In a few instances, surgery can be required to remove broken tissue or improve blood flow to the affected location. Surgical options for stress ulcers can encompass debridement, pores and skin grafts, and tissue flaps. These approaches can be complex and may require a lengthy healing time, so working closely with a healthcare provider is critical to determine if surgical treatment is the best alternative for your situation.

Stopping stress ulcers is always a pleasant course of action, and this may be completed by taking steps to lessen stress in the pores, skin, and underlying tissue. People at risk for stress ulcers have to be repositioned often, and they ought to be furnished with supportive cushions or mattresses to reduce strain on the pores and skin. Top vitamins are likewise critical for stopping stress ulcers, as a healthy eating regimen can help improve skin health and promote restoration.

Pressure ulcers are an extreme fitness concern that could cause vast headaches if left untreated. Happily, there are numerous specific remedy options to be had for people who are suffering from stress ulcers. Whether you are using dressings, topical retailers, or a surgical operation, working closely with a healthcare provider is crucial to decide the satisfactory course of action for your individual state of affairs. And don't forget, prevention is always the best alternative about pressure ulcers, so take steps to lessen stress on the pores and skin and maintain good nutrition to keep your pores and skin healthy and sturdy.

Pressure ulcers, also called bedsores or pressure sores, are commonplace for folks who are bedridden or have restricted mobility. Those sores are due to prolonged strain on the pores and skin, which could cause tissue harm or contamination. If left untreated, pressure ulcers can be painful and might even bring about extreme fitness issues. Happily, there are numerous unique treatment alternatives for pressure ulcers, depending on the severity of the sore and the man's or women normal health. One of the most common remedies for strain ulcers is converting positions more regularly. This will help alleviate the strain on the affected area and allow the skin to heal. For people who are bedridden or have restricted mobility, this may include using a unique bed or cushion to distribute their weight more evenly and reduce strain on certain regions. To prevent skin irritation, keeping the location clean and dry and using a barrier cream to shield the skin is important.

In more extreme instances, surgical intervention can be necessary. This will involve draining any pus or fluid collected inside the store or removing any lifeless tissue. Pores and skin grafts can also promote recovery and save you from infection.

Every other remedy alternative for pressure ulcers involves the use of topical remedies, together with hydro gels or dressings. These treatments can help reduce pain and infection and restore the pores and skin. Some topical remedies also assist in keeping the wound wet, which may help promote restoration.

Further to these treatment options, many healthcare providers may recommend particular nutritional and hydration interventions to facilitate healing. Consuming a properly balanced weight-reduction plan rich in protein and nutrients can help promote skin health and boost healing.

It is critical to note that prevention is usually the best course of action regarding stress ulcers. Avoiding prolonged stress on the skin, preserving proper hygiene, and staying properly nourished and hydrated can all help to prevent the development of stress ulcers in the first place.

Strain ulcers can be a painful and critical problem, but numerous treatment options are available depending on the severity of the sore and the patient's general fitness. Changing positions regularly, topical treatments, and surgical intervention are all possible options. However, prevention remains the best way to avoid pressure ulcers altogether. Individuals can substantially reduce their risk of developing strain ulcers by practicing good hygiene, staying well-nourished and hydrated, and avoiding extended stress on the pores and skin.

CHAPTER FIVE

COMPLICATIONS OF PRESSURE ULCERS

Pressure ulcers, also called bedsores or strain sores, are a not unusual medical condition that can have full-size complications if left untreated. These sores broaden while some of the skin is subjected to constant strain, especially in those who are bedridden or have restricted mobility. we can discover the complications of pressure ulcers and why it's essential to seek clinical attention immediately.

Hardship #1: infection

One of the most critical complications of pressure ulcers is contamination. When the pores and skin are broken, they become prone to microorganisms. If left untreated, these infections can spread to different elements of the body, consisting of the bones, blood, and inner organs. The risk of contamination increases with the severity of the pressure ulcer. In some instances, sepsis, a life-threatening situation, can broaden.

Problem #2: behind schedule restoration

If left untreated, stress ulcers can take a long time to heal. This is due to the fact that the body's natural recovery method is bogged down by the non-stop stress in the affected area. In some instances, the ulcer might also by no means heal completely, leading to a chronic wound that calls for ongoing treatment.

Complication #3: Muscle and bone harm

Pressure ulcers can harm the underlying muscular tissues and bones. This can lead to a loss of muscles and strength, as well as bone fractures and other bone-related complications. In intense instances, surgery may be required to restore the damage.

Problem #4: reduced quality of life

Pressure ulcers can be extremely painful and uncomfortable, making it tough for sufferers to perform their primary daily tasks or experience their hobbies. They can also result in social isolation and melancholy, as sufferers may feel ashamed or embarrassed about their condition.

Difficulty #5: Accelerated Healthcare Costs

The treatment of stress ulcers can be expensive, specifically if the circumstances have progressed to an intense level. Patients can also require hospitalization, a surgical operation, or long-term period care, all of which may be luxurious.

Further, the cost of treating headaches and infections can similarly drive up healthcare expenses.

Pressure ulcers are a serious medical condition that can cause great headaches if left untreated. Infections, not-on-time recuperation, muscle and bone damage, reduced satisfaction of existence, and increased healthcare fees are just a few of the capability headaches. In case you or a loved one is vulnerable to developing strain ulcers, it's vital to take preventative measures and seek scientific attention right away if you notice any signs of skin breakdown. With the right care and remedy, many of those complications may be avoided.

Dialogue about the complications that may arise if stress ulcers are not treated nicely

Pressure ulcers, also called bedsores, are not uncommon trouble for folks who are restricted to a mattress or wheelchair for prolonged durations. Those ulcers can cause a tremendous deal of pain, soreness, and even severe headaches if left untreated. In this newsletter, we will discuss the complications that may arise if pressure ulcers are not dealt with well. First and foremost, pressure ulcers can result in infections. This happens when the skin around the ulcer becomes damaged, permitting microorganisms to enter the body. If left untreated, those infections can spread to different parts of the body, leading to sepsis or other lifestyle-threatening situations.

Additionally, stress ulcers can cause huge pain and suffering. The regular strain on the affected area can cause nerve damage, making movement and even sitting difficult. This ache can be particularly debilitating for elderly individuals or those with present fitness conditions.

Another hassle associated with pressure ulcers is the development of deep tissue and bone infections. When stress ulcers are left untreated, they are able to start to have an effect on the deeper layers of tissue and even the bone. This could cause severe infections, which might be difficult to deal with and may require surgical treatment to remove inflamed tissue.

In some cases, strain ulcers can also lead to the development of gangrene. Gangrene occurs when tissue dies because of a loss of blood flow, and it could be a life-threatening situation. If a strain ulcer is left untreated for a long period of time, it is able to ultimately cause the improvement of gangrene within the affected region.

Subsequently, stress ulcers can also contribute to the overall decline in a person's fitness and well-being. The constant pain associated with stress ulcers can cause depression, tension, and different intellectual health issues. These, in turn, can make it even more difficult for individuals to get over the ulcers and regain their health. Strain ulcers are a severe problem that can lead to huge headaches if left untreated. If you or a loved one is at risk for developing strain ulcers, it's critical to take steps to prevent them from happening in the first place. This can include normal repositioning, the use of special cushions or mattresses, and other measures to reduce strain on the skin. If a strain ulcer does develop, it's important to seek clinical attention as quickly as possible to prevent additional complications from arising.

Pressure ulcers, additionally known as bedsores or stress sores, are not unusual situations that can have an effect on anybody who spends extended periods of time in bed or motionless. These ulcers are due to prolonged stress on the pores and skin and may cause great pain if left untreated. If stress ulcers are not treated well, they can result in quite a number of complications that can have serious effects on someone's fitness and well-being. One of the biggest headaches associated with untreated pressure ulcers is infection. When the skin is broken with the aid of a pressure ulcer, it will become more susceptible to microorganisms and other pathogens that could cause infections. If contamination takes hold, it may unfold quickly and even cause sepsis, a life-threatening circumstance that could cause organ failure and other extreme health problems. In addition to the danger of contamination, strain ulcers can also cause widespread aches and pains that make it difficult for someone to sleep, eat, or perform daily sports.

Another worry about untreated strain ulcers is damage to the underlying tissue and bones. As pressure ulcers progress, they can cause damage to the deeper layers of pores, skin, and tissue, eventually reaching the bone. This will result in the development of osteomyelitis, a critical bone contamination that can be tough to deal with and might require surgical treatment. In severe cases, this will cause amputation of the affected limb.

Stress ulcers can also have a vast effect on a person's intellectual health and well-being. Many human beings with pressure ulcers experience feelings of disgrace, embarrassment, and social isolation that could lead to melancholy and tension. In addition, the pain and soreness associated with pressure ulcers can make it difficult for a person to have interaction in sports they revel in or preserve social connections, which could similarly exacerbate feelings of isolation and loneliness.

Sooner or later, untreated pressure ulcers can lead to longer clinic stays and increased healthcare fees. If a stress ulcer becomes inflamed or results in different headaches, a person may additionally want to stay in a medical institution for a prolonged period of time to obtain treatment. This could be costly and also disrupt someone's day-to-day routine.

Pressure ulcers are a common condition that could have tremendous outcomes if left untreated. If you or a loved one is experiencing pressure ulcers, it's crucial to search for clinical interest as quickly as possible to ensure proper treatment and avoid potential headaches. With proper care and attention, stress ulcers can be correctly managed, and the chance of headaches may be minimized, allowing people to maintain their fitness, well-being, and high quality of life.

CONCLUSION OF PRESSURE ULCERS

Strain ulcers are a common hassle that affects many humans. These sores can increase on the skin over bony areas of the frame, such as the hips, heels, and tailbone, because of extended stress or friction. They may be particularly common in individuals who are immobile or bedridden, such as the elderly or critically Even though pressure ulcers can be painful and difficult to manage, there are numerous steps you can take to prevent them and ensure recovery if they do occur. Step one in preventing pressure ulcers is to recognize those who are at risk. This consists of those who are bedridden, have decreased sensation, have poor vitamins, or have medical situations that affect circulation. For these individuals, it's vital to take steps to relieve strain on bony regions of the frame, along with changing positions often, using unique cushions or mattresses, and warding off tight clothing or bedding. Different measures that could help save you from strain ulcers consist of maintaining exact hygiene, keeping the pores and skin moisturized, and providing good vitamins and hydration.

If stress ulcers do occur, it's critical to initiate treatment as soon as possible to promote healing and prevent similar harm. This can include cleaning the wound and masking it with a sterile dressing, the use of medications or lotions to promote recovery, and imparting pain relief as desired. In some cases, surgery can be important to repair damaged tissue or restore underlying structures.

The lengthy-term management of strain ulcers includes ongoing monitoring and preventive measures to prevent recurrence. This could consist of regular pores and skin checks, using suitable strain-relieving devices, imparting good enough vitamins and hydration, and selling mobility and interest as appropriate.

Strain ulcers are a commonplace hassle that can be averted and controlled with proper care and interest. By figuring out people by chance, taking preventive measures, and presenting active treatment while needed, it's far more viable to sell recovery and save you similar harm. With ongoing management and monitoring, individuals with stress ulcers can revel in a satisfactory lifestyle and avoid the complications that can result from this condition.

Strain ulcers, additionally known as bedsores or strain sores, are a commonplace problem for those who are bedridden or have restrained mobility. These sores can vary from slight to excessive and might cause widespread pain and ache for those affected. we will talk about the importance of preventing stress ulcers and the steps you can take to avoid them. Prevention is key when it comes to stress ulcers. Step one in preventing stress ulcers is to maintain correct hygiene and skin care. This means regularly cleaning and moisturizing the pores and skin, in addition to ensuring that any incontinence problems are immediately addressed. It's also important to avoid excessive moisture, as this will weaken the pores and skin and increase the risk of damage.

Another essential way to prevent stress ulcers is to reposition the body regularly. This indicates changing positions often, mainly for folks who are bedridden or have confined mobility. This may assist in alleviating stress on inclined areas of the body, which include the hips, heels, and again. It is also crucial to use proper positioning strategies, together with the use of pillows or supports, to maintain the body in the appropriate alignment.

Similarly to those preventative measures, there are also several treatment alternatives to be had for those who have already developed pressure ulcers. Remedy alternatives might also consist of the use of specialized cushions or mattresses, wound dressings, and antibiotics to prevent infection. In severe cases, surgery can be important to dispose of damaged tissue or provide recuperation. In the long run, the important thing to do to stop pressure ulcers is to be proactive and take the necessary steps to preserve proper skin hygiene and reduce stress on susceptible regions of the body. By doing so, you can help to avoid the development of these painful and doubtless extreme sores and preserve your basic fitness and wellness.

Strain ulcers are a not uncommon trouble that can cause vast discomfort and ache for those affected. However, by taking a proactive approach to skincare and frequently repositioning the frame, you can help prevent the development of those sores and maintain your fitness and well-being.

THE END

Milton Keynes UK
Ingram Content Group UK Ltd.
UKHW031833300124
436988UK00013B/856